Body Makeover in 4 Hours

How to Get Bigger, Leaner, & Stay Healthier Longer

By Cathy Wilson
Copyright © 2013

Income Disclaimer

This book contains business strategies, marketing methods and other business advice that, regardless of my own results and experience, may not produce the same results (or any results) for you. I make absolutely no guarantee, expressed or implied, that by following the advice below you will make any money or improve current profits, as there are several factors and variables that come into play regarding any given business.

Primarily, results will depend on the nature of the product or business model, the conditions of the marketplace, the experience of the individual, and situations and elements that are beyond your control.

As with any business endeavor, you assume all risk related to investment and money based on your own discretion and at your own potential expense.

Liability Disclaimer

By reading this book, you assume all risks associated with using the advice given below, with a full understanding that you, solely, are responsible for anything that may occur as a result of putting this information into action in any way, and regardless of your interpretation of the advice.

You further agree that our company cannot be held responsible in any way for the success or failure of your business as a result of the information presented in this book. It is your responsibility to conduct your own due diligence regarding the safe and successful operation of

your business if you intend to apply any of our information in any way to your business operations.

Terms of Use

You are given a non-transferable, "personal use" license
to this book. You cannot distribute it or share it with other
individuals.

Also, there are no resale rights or private label rights
granted when purchasing this book. In other words, it's
for your own personal use only.

Body Makeover in 4 Hours

How to Get Bigger, Leaner, & Stay Healthier Longer

By Cathy Wilson

Table of Contents

Introduction

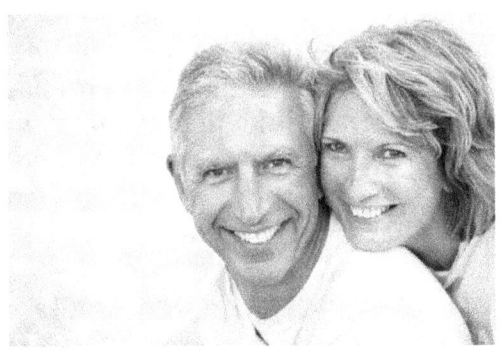

This is NOT, The 4 Hour Body book. It's the Body Make-over in 4 Hours: How to Get Bigger, Leaner, & Healthier.

This is not a magical weight loss book where at the end of your reading I give you some magical beans in a "special limited time offer of just 12 easy installments of $19.95 if you act now!" It isn't where I fill your noggin full of lead and promise you with little or no effort you get to eat anything you want and you're GUARANTEED to lose 20 pounds of FAT in the first week and keep it off forever! Sorry to disappoint you.

I think to some degree we've all "been there-done that." I am passionate about health and wellness. I am always looking to better myself one step at a time. With over 20 years studying and researching health and wellness, writing numerous books and working with lots of expert medical professionals in various fields of health and wellness, I have come to understand what "good" health is all about.

It's multi-factorial and different for each one of us. You need to educate yourself on the basics and take with you the bits and pieces from each health strategy you learn and use what works for you. Consider your preferences and tolerances and take what "fits" you. It's never about finding the "perfect" eating strategy or exercise program. It's about diversity always, figuring out what works for you and always looking to better it. Right or wrong is the furthest from what this is about. Focus on "bettering you" and you're off to the races.

This Body Makeover in 4 Hours is all about . . .

* Using healthy eating strategies, similar to the infamous Paleo "caveman" natural eating still that's been hogging the spotlight lately.

* Understanding and brainstorming to incorporate regular intense physical activity into your day, just like people have done since the beginning of time.

* Adding the importance of preventing disease and dealing with health issues on the table instead of bandaging them and wishing them away, just like you do taking a tablet for a headache, migraine or TMJ pain.

* Recognizing how important sleep in is your health and making sure sleep issues are dealt with and strategies are put in place to get the quality and quantity of sleep your body needs to recharge.

PLUS:

* Making sure you take care of the mental. Your mind and body need to work as one if you are going to build your body bigger, leaner, stronger, and longer. The mind is a powerful thing and if you learn how to take care it,

and you'll be surprised how quickly your life will turn, positively at that.

So, what's the 4 Hour Body connection? Without getting too technical, let me talk a little about 4 Hour Body Theory. This uncommon weight loss, muscle building plan focuses on fast weight-loss, awesome sex and transforming superhuman holds a lot of useful strategies for bettering health as a whole. This issue is that it's VERY extreme and it really doesn't matter if something is "scientifically" possible if it's not practical.

Let's face it. Most of us have issues making the switch as simple as white bread to brown. The expectation is a super short intense amount of time with this "4 Hour Body" is pretty unrealistic for most of us. By taking the "good" out of this health and wellness strategy and adding some practicality and addressing a few more essential factors in good health, you will have a solid base from which to build your new healthy life habits that will help you . . .

* Lose weight fast and keep it off
* Gain energy and optimism
* Strengthen your immune system and deter disease
* Lessen chronic and painful symptoms
* Improve your cognitive capacity
* Strengthen self-confidence and life satisfaction

LONG-TERM!

With only 4 hours a week of muscle building and cardiovascular training you can build your body bigger, leaner, stronger, and longer, helping to boost your metabolism and burn fat, releasing stress, gaining energy, deterring disease, boosting your spirit and so much more. That's just over 30 minutes per day!

This isn't about bandaging life issues that get you down, but rather finding solutions that work for you and applying them to the best or your abilities. Any change is good change. It's one foot in front of the other all eyes forward. Never quit, always persist and you WILL reach your goals and I will show you how.

In Days Past

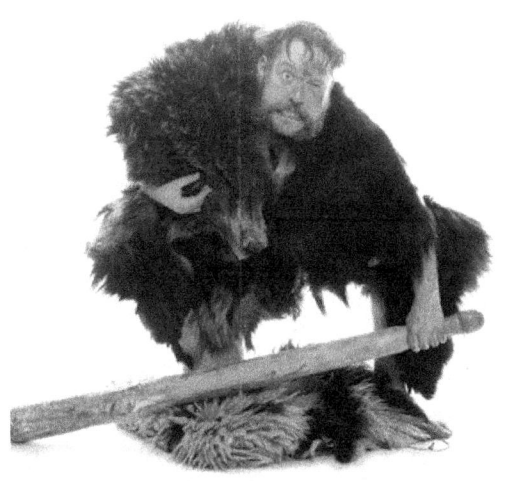

We are in constant motion, always changing, a constant since the beginning of time. Experts have evidence our genes are nutritionally interconnected with our ancestors of the Paleolithic era some 2.5 billion years past. Digging further into this, scientists believe they will uncover clues to help understand better the diseases and food imbalances that stress us today.

The Paleolithic or "hunter-gatherer" period ended about 10,000 years ago when agriculture was introduced. It's believed people from this Paleolithic time ate mainly foods hunted or fished, including a wide range of wild game, fish and other seafood. This was where they got their muscle building and energy triggering protein, an essential macronutrient needed for survival.

Protein isn't made by the body nor is it stored, so it's important to eat it at least 2-3 times per day. Our ancestors had it right. Fish and seafood served up protective omega 3 and 6 fatty acids, helping protect against skin conditions, cancers, diabetes, and heart problems. Omega 9 is the fatty acid produced by the body if 3 and 6 are present. So healthy fats, vital protein and other essential vitamins and minerals the body requires to function optimally were covered by hunting.

The rest of their nutrition was made up with the "gathering" of foods. Carbohydrates, vitamins and minerals were satisfied with these foods. Examples are such things as plants, nuts, herbs, spices, nuts, fresh berries and fruits, eggs, mushrooms, other fungi and insects.

These people ate only what natured offered because there was no other option. They were extremely physical because their very survival depended on it. No couches or soda and chip parties for our ancestors. They threw a party when they had enough food to eat, all-natural organic food straight from Mother Nature to their tummy.

Nutrition

To eat thousands of years ago required people, or at least the hunters, to be in tip-top shape. Diets were mainly lean meats of antelope, wildebeest, gazelles and whatever game was available in the region. This meant diets varied considerably from place to place and people had no choice but to adapt. If the food supply was running thin for any reasons; disease, drought or perhaps flooding, villages and communities had to move elsewhere to find the meat they needed to survive.

Often the hunters would track down and go after the weakest link in the herd. A young calf, one that was injured, and older animals that we already in the stages of dying, were the frequently the "chosen" ones.

Meat gave the nutritional protein required to keep the mind sharp, muscles strong and healthy, energy levels up, and meat was easier on the digestive system. Scientists believe lean meats were critical in fueling the brain to grow and advance.

Of course meats lack dietary fiber which is essential in proper growth, development and bodily function. Various fruits, plants, nuts, seeds, herbs and spices made up the remainder of all-natural and wholesome diet of our ancestors. This is where other macronutrients including carbohydrates for longer term energy and good fats, for energy, organ protection and brain function came into play. These macronutrients are needed in large amounts and are essential because your body doesn't make them, so they must be eaten.

Other vital nutrients provided from these "gathering" foods are:

Fiber - rids the body of waste
Potassium - critical for proper function of nerves, muscles, kidney and heart health
Folate - helps prevent osteoporosis, depressions and helps with development
Vitamin A - important in eye and skin health, improves resistance to infection
Vitamin C - healthy skin helps with gum and teeth health and with nutrient absorption
These are just a few of the nutrients your body needs to support its internal systems and function optimally. Lacking in any one micronutrient can trigger disease and illness.

Exercise

People didn't have a choice here. Either they were in excellent physical condition or they didn't survive. The strongest survived and that was just a reality in days past. Physical was required for all the necessities of life; shelter, food, clothing and water.

Illness/Disease

If your body wasn't strong enough to fight off disease you would die. The only medicines per say available were natural and holistic, many of which were no match for serious disease that wiped out whole communities in one foul swoop. Staying fit and eating healthy was the only defense these people had when sickness surfaced, for the most part anyway.

Sleep

Our ancestors understood better and listened to their bodies closer, or so it seems. Experts agree our ancestors, way back in time routinely got about 8 hours of sleep on average. The body's mental and physical need to shut down completely and regenerate. The only time this can be done is with sleep, an undisturbed quality sleep that's going to give the mind and body a rest so they can function optimally the next day.

Mental

Mental alertness was top priority for people from times past. Their very survival depended on it. The physical exercise helped relieve stress, relax and sharpen the mental. During the day their minds were always working, meaning they did well with the "you snooze, you lose" theory. Exercising the mind was a given in this world.

My Thoughts . . .

Our ancestors may have had it tough, but the sure lived healthy, natural, adventurous lives. They listened to their bodies, had little interference and had no choice but to battle the perils of nature; weather, disease and natural disaster. Fittest of the fit was reality and the conveniences of our society today wasn't an option. Can you even imagine?

Reality of Life Today

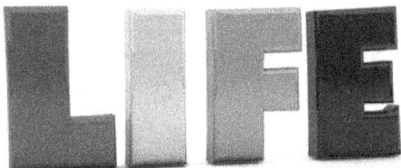

Boy, have we done a good job screwing up or internal bodily systems, causing extreme stress and interferences that encourage chronic conditions, disease, sickness and various debilitating ailments that take away directly from our quality of life. Our physical, emotional, mental and lifestyle as a whole suffers.

The idea of progress sounds positive, but with it, comes the price of good health. We want convenience and this means processed fatty foods high in bad fats with little nutritional value. We have created such a stressful environment trying to fit everything in and forcing our good health to pay the price.

* Less sleep is now a constant in most people's lives.

* Desk jobs with lots of button pushing is the norm. Little if any, physical exercise occurs.

* Our world revolves around money and greed. Who can make the most by giving the least, regardless of the price

to paycheck. Manufacturers produce foods to stock the shelves with nutrition-less fuel in pretty packaging with dangerous Trans fat because they are cheaper and give a longer shelf life. There has to be something wrong with "meats" that last a month?

* With advanced industrial production, come increased environmental toxins. Each seep at some point into our natural ecosystem, the waters, into the soil and into food, the animals we eat are tainted with poison. With every action is a reaction and for your body and health the re-action does not look very promising.

* The mental stress we create for ourselves is very dangerous. Centuries ago the regular physical reality of each day was enough to satisfy stress, the natural physical "fight or flight" response to stressful stimuli, an automated response. When presented with this "stress" today, we might decide to take a nap or drown our depression with a big tub of ice cream on the couch.

We have systematically and habitually removed the "physical" the body is programmed to use when dealing with stressful stimuli and this means toxic buildup. Over time these stresses will transform into disease, sickness and illness, both mental and physical, causing further breakdown of good health.

By eating poorly, poisoning our environment, starving our bodies of sleep regularly, not de-stressing and building our minds and bodies strong with regular physical exercise and ignoring our "mental" needs, we are literally destroying our quality and quantity of life.

Insane - Is all about continuing with the same actions and expecting different results.

Change - Something humans tend to shy away from because we are creatures of habit and find comfort in
routine, good or bad.

You choose. Are you ready to make some reasonable
and sustainable positive health changes for the better, or
would you rather make excuses and continue on your
downward spiral?

Nutrition

What have we done to healthy eating? By creating unhealthy eating patterns, we have programmed our taste
buds to crave refined sugars and high-fat foods with very
little nutritional value.

***Did You Know . . . By grabbing a sweet treat to tie
your hunger over till dinner, you are actually teaching your body to crave sweets whenever you are
"really" hungry. It's best to eat healthy foods when
hungry and if you still crave something sweet have it
in moderation. Doing this will keep you from caving
to sweet cravings when your resistance is down because your tummy is empty.***

With fast-food restaurants on every corner it's just too
convenient to grab something on the way home from
work rather than take the time to cook a nutritious and
wholesome meal. Social pressures to indulge appear
during the holidays, birthdays and when friends get together to let off steam. Birds of a feather flock together.
When one person decides to have another beer and
plate of chicken wings it's like the stamp of approval for
everyone else, regardless of whether anyone is hungry or
not.

We have taught ourselves to eat for emotional reasons. When we feel depressed a bag of chips and a soda will temporarily boost our spirits. When celebrating, it's like we just received a ticket to pig-out without consequence. Getting together with friends and family almost always encircles drink and food, and rarely the healthy versions. Our poor eating habits cause obesity and a whole whack of other serious health issues. They interfere with our energy, good sleep, strong body and mind and poor eating leaves us feeling defeated and depressed. Sound familiar?

Exercise

Exercise? What are you talking about? I walked to get the mail 3 times last week!

The mind is a powerful thing and you can pretty much find justification in anything you do if that's what you actually think and believe. Exercise takes effort. REAL exercise works your heart and lungs for extended periods of time and your will be sweating before you're through. The problem here is most of us have got stuck in the cycle of not exercising and this means we are going to have to get our head into the game before the body will follow.

FACT - *Your body needs exercise every single day to stay strong for you. To keep you lean and strong, deter disease, avoid chronic aches and pains, keep your mind sharp and to give you the energy you need to make the most of every day. If you choose to not give your body the cardiovascular and muscular exercise it requires, then over time you will lose your mobility and mobility and eventually you are going to be at the mercy of your poor health. PREVENTION is the key and regular physical exercise, the kind that requires REAL effort is critical.*

Your body needs both cardiovascular and weight training/strength training. Starting with 30 minutes cardiovascular 3-5 days a week and 15 minutes weight or strength training 2-3 times a week is a good base. Of course you should always start slow and run it by your physician first. The guidance of a fitness trainer is always a good idea to set you up for success, a good one will have a look at your abilities, health issues, preferences and tolerances, weight loss goals, among other factors and create a personalized plan for you. After a short time, you should be able to take this base and build on it yourself if you'd like.

Keep in mind anything is better than nothing. If you can only start with 15 minutes of heart pumping activity, a brisk walk around the block, then that's great. It's got to "fit" you. It's trial and error.

Illness/Disease

* Almost a million people die from cardiovascular disease each year.

* Experts suggest over 90% of disease is triggered or complicated because of stress.

* Studies show every 3 minutes a woman is diagnosed officially with breast cancer.

A disease is simply an abnormal condition which directly affects the function of an organism. Over time serious disease and illness has manifested and scientific researchers believe this is due to numerous factors, including . . .

* Toxic chemicals we create that infiltrate our environment, water, food and world in which we live.

* Viruses have developed resistance to medicines.

* Our unhealthy lifestyles decrease or resistance to disease.

Sleep

Over time with progress and technological advancements
we have created more interference with the connection
between mind and body. If we aren't "listening" to our
body when it comes to sleep, we are then creating negative sleep habits. For instance, if we are working late and
start to feel tired, we might grab a cup of coffee to syn-
thetically wake ourselves up to work later, interfering with
our natural sleep cycle which short circuits our hormone
function, sleep rhythm and functioning of our body as a
whole.

We've come to accept the fact that less sleep is neces-
sary in our world today and by depriving ourselves of
sleep we are only increasing bodily stresses. This has
dire consequences for our health, both mental and physical.

Mental

The mental is often left out of healthy eating and exercising strategies, when really it should be priority one. If you
head isn't on board with all these positive lifestyle changes your chance so long-term success is just about
obsolete!

My Thoughts . . .

*It really can be depressing looking at the obvious causal
factors for many of our health issues. It's US that have
created the issues. Flipping to the positive, this just*

means that you and I need to make the changes to make things better. By accepting, gaining knowledge and taking positive action you can grab hold of good health long-term and reel it in.

The 4 PLUS - Nutrition, Exercise, Ill- ness/Disease, Sleep, Mental

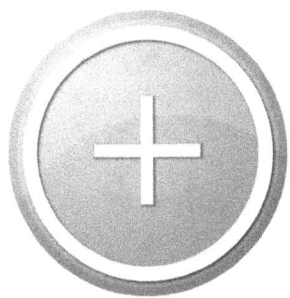

Nutrition

By definition nutrition is the process of supplying food to an organism in order to keep it alive. If you are incorporating the science of it all, it's the practice of eating and utilizing the nutrients in foods.

When it comes to nutrition you are what you eat! By eating healthy with plenty of lean meat, health carbohydrates, good fats and essential vitamins and minerals your body requires for optimal function, you will build your body and mind bigger, leaner, stronger, longer. Nutrition is also about disease and condition prevention through proper diet.

The 7 main nutrients you need for a healthy body are:

* Protein (2-3 servings/day)
* Carbohydrates (5-6 servings/day)

* Fats (2-3 servings)
* Vitamins
* Minerals
* Water (6-8 glasses)
* Antioxidants

Protein

Every single cell in your body has protein. Protein is a macronutrient that's essential, meaning it isn't found in your body and you need it in large amounts.

The technical functions of proteins are:

* Triggering various internal chemical reactions
* Form cells structures within cells
* Fight disease and illness
* Transfer vital nutrients throughout the body
* Act as the director of cell function

The amounts of protein you need is dependent on your:
- Activity level
- Body composition
- Weight and height
- Age
- Health
- Total calories consumed

If you don't get adequate protein into your body daily you can experience

- Skin dullness
- Hair loss and extreme tiredness
- Muscle loss
- Trouble concentrating
- Poor memory
- Hormone issues

- Fertility problems
- Decreased sex drive
- Moodiness

Some of the issues today are that we often get **too much** protein and the **wrong** kind. Eating breaded deep fried chicken, processed meats like hot dogs and luncheon meats, canned meats like Spam, butter pan-fried fatty meats and Trans fat loaded fast food beef and chicken is just going to get you into trouble.

These are all loaded with bad "saturated" fats, high salt and lots of calories. A portion of protein is the size of a deck of cards or 3/4s a cup of beans or 1/3 cup of nuts for reference, which is a heck of a lot less than even one restaurant serving. A chicken sandwich or burger is usually 2-3 servings of unhealthy protein at one sitting!

Consequence of Too Much Protein
* Increased toxins which can result in liver issues
* Protein in your urine - associated with diabetes
* Bone weakening because of interference in calcium absorption
* Increase in adult-onset diabetes
* Weakening of immune system
* Obesity, gaining weight

Reasons Proteins are Important for Good Health

Amino acids are essential to life and without protein these amino acids can't be broken down and utilized. The foods you eat with AA offers up the missing amino acids, the building blocks of life.

Protein is energy and a part of every cell in your body, making it very important to supply your body with it every day.

Some very good sources of protein are: lean beef, skinless chicken, turkey and other protein, beans, eggs, nuts, dairy products, whole grains, fish and seafood, soy

Carbohydrates

Essentially your body uses carbohydrates to create glucose which is what gives your body energy to function. Carbohydrates can be stored or used immediately.

2 Kinds:

Complex

These are the carbs your body wants, whole grain breads, whole wheat pasta, brown rice, beans and vegetables. They also contain dietary fiber, essential in getting rid of harmful toxins in your system.

SOLUBLE FIBER is found in foods like:

* Seeds and nuts
* Many fruits, oatmeal and beans
* Peas and oat bran

INSOLUBLE FIBER is found in foods including:
* Whole grain breads and cereals
* Seeds and vegetables
* Fruits
* Couscous, brown rice and pasta

Simple

These carbs give you quick energy, but it doesn't last. It's just like a shot of adrenaline and then your energy levels drop into the basement fast. White breads, pastas, rice, pastries and other sweets are going to give your body short-term energy with little or no nutritional value, giving you a shot of sugar that pushes your blood sugar through the roof, only to have it plummet into despair shortly after. Simple carbohydrates are often chemically modified sugars that increase your risk of obesity and developing serious disease like diabetes for one. Chances are pretty good if you're a junk-food-junkie you are eating mainly simple sugars and your body and mind are paying the price.

By making the choice to avoid bad carbs and incorporate healthy complex carbohydrate foods into your diet, 4-6 servings every day, you will provide your body with the energy and vital macronutrient to overall good health.

Fats

Fats are what seem to get us into loads of trouble health-wise. Many don't understand there is a big difference between a healthy (unsaturated) fat and an unhealthy (saturated or Trans) fat.

Experts agree that less than 25% of your daily caloric intake should come from fat, closer to 20% is ideal.

Saturated/Trans Fat

These fats are what you want to stay away from for the most part. They are found in sweet and tasty processed foods and animal products like meat and dairy products. These fats aren't good for your health and are recognized for raising cholesterol levels.

Obesity is linked directly with the overconsumption of these fats, particularly with fast-foods, convenience foods that are boxed, packaged and have a long shelf life. Just think pastries, cookies, muffins, chips, chocolate bars and other sweets.

Not only do these types of foods make us fat, but they also poison our systems with loads of chemicals and preservatives we can't digest. Over time these toxins build up and interfere with the smooth function of our internal systems,.causing all sorts of health complications that may surface first as mild conditions, only later to manifest into serious disease that kills.

* Saturated fats should be avoided because they are only going to harm your body function, causing extreme fatigue, sleep issues, moodiness, increased disease, heart disease, stroke, diabetes, decreased cognitive capacity to start. Instead choose healthy fats in moderation and you will get do your mind and body a favor.

* Unsaturated Fats are what you want to eat. Avocados, nuts and olives are great sources. These fats are liquid at room temperature and experts deem them "heart healthy." They can actually help lower bad cholesterol and raise good cholesterol.

Healthy fat is needed for survival. You need fat for energy, protecting your major organs and to provide your body with fat-soluble vitamins. Eating fat in your diet is the only way you can get the two essential fatty acids that will help in the formation of cell membranes, vision and healthy immune system function.

What's important to note here, is that our problem as a society is that we eat too much fat as a whole, both saturated and unsaturated. In order to lose weight, construct lean muscle and build your body strong, you need to lower your daily fat intake and make sure you are getting just enough for your bodily systems to function. The fact remains it really doesn't matter what you are eating. If you are consuming too much you are going to get fat and this will interfere with all of your bodily systems, mind and body.

Vitamins and Minerals, Water and Antioxidants

Vitamins are made by plants or animals and minerals are simply inorganic elements derived from the earth. In order for your body to grow and develop normally you need essential vitamins in minerals or micronutrients in small amounts.

Some common vitamins and minerals are:

- Chromium, calcium and folate
- Iron, selenium and magnesium
- Vitamin A, B6, B12, D, E and K
- Zinc

Your body needs Vitamin D to help build strong bones, healthy hair and skin and also to increase the absorption of calcium. If you neglect to get enough Vitamin D your bones can soften (rickets) because you aren't absorbing enough calcium. Your body doesn't make calcium so this is an essential vitamin and you need to get it through your diet. The best route to getting your vitamins and minerals is to eat a healthy diet full of lean meats and plenty of fresh fruits and vegetables and mineral amounts of good fats. You can get your calcium either from plant or milk sources.

Water is also something you need to survive. Every living organism needs water. You can probably go a week without food, but wouldn't last more than a day or two without water.

Others Reasons to Drink Water

* Your body is two-thirds water - Muscle is up to 70% water and is what powers your body. If you are dehydrated your body gets stressed and can't function.

* Helps transport vital nutrients to your tissues and vital organs

* Regulates body temperature

* Helps internal chemical reactions

* Lubricates joints and intricate systems

* Keeps skin from drying

* Gives you energy

* Helps regulate bowel movements

* Improves immunity by keeping your lungs, mucous membranes and sinus passages from getting dried out
* Helps with weight loss because a hydrated body has higher levels of oxygen in the bloodstream. This means your body is more efficiently burning fat.

6-8 glasses of water each day is something everyone should strive for. Of course if you are exercising more or happen to live in a warmer climate, you will have to up your water intake.

Antioxidants are essentially natural compounds in specific foods that help protect the body from disease by neutralizing dangerous free-radicals. Free-radicals are naturally occurring substances in your body that attack

34

your cells, fast-forwarding the aging process and triggering disease.

Great Sources of Antioxidants

Blueberries
Blackberries
Raspberries
Broccoli
Apples
Spinach
Cabbage
Beans
Green Tea
Red Wine
Dark chocolate
Red, orange, yellow peppers

Fruits and vegetables that are brightly colored are often loaded with these powerful protective antioxidants that are great for your health.

Note: It does not matter where you begin here. Maybe you think a French fry is a vegetable and don't think you could make it around the block without needing an oxygen tank. SO WHAT!

What matters is you make the decision and commitment to change things, to work on your eating and learning to fit physical exercise into your every day. There are no shortcuts here and everyone has to start from ground zero at some point. There's no use measuring where you aren't. How about looking at where you are today and making a plan to move ahead one step at a time, considering your preferences and tolerances, to better long-term health overall?

Serving Sizes Explained!

So many of us, are in fantasy land when it comes to serving sizes. We think the plate in front of us at a restaurant is what our body needs, which is completely crazy because most restaurant servings are 2-3 times the size your body needs to run. Here are the basics of serving sizes so you can make sure you aren't over or under-eating with your portions.

MEAT AND MEAT PRODUCTS

Meats - approximately the size of a deck of cards
Beans - two-thirds of a cup
Eggs - 1-2
Nuts - 1/3 cup
Peanut Butter - 1-2 tablespoons

BREADS AND CEREALS
Bread - 1 slice
Bagel - 1/2 bagel
Oatmeal - 1/2-2/4 cup
Cereals - 1/2-3/4 cup
Pasta/Rice - 3/4 cup

MILK AND MILK PRODUCTS
Milk - 1 cup
Yogurt - 1/2 cup
Cottage Cheese - 1/2 cup
Cheese - 2x2 inch cube

FRUITS AND VEGETABLES
Whole Fruit - 1
Fruit - 3/4 cup
Vegetables - 3/4 cup
Dried Fruit - 2-3 tablespoons

HEALTHY FATS
Oils - 1-2 tablespoons
Avocado - 1/4 cup

Note - various healthy foods are loaded with healthy fats, like nuts and various seeds. Most people don't have to look to add fat into their diet but concentrate on making sure they are eating the right fat in reduced amounts.

Exercise

Most people have conditioned themselves to have a love or hate relationship with exercise and studies show that most overweight or obese people have convinced themselves to hate exercise for whatever reasons. Somewhere along the path of life we've taught ourselves to become lazy and disconnect with our body with regards to eating right, exercising and taking care of our mental wellness.

I can't stop you from making excuses to exercise or not, but I can tell you that your body, just the same as your ancestors, was programmed and built for exercising regularly. Routing physical activity will keep your mind and body strong, keep disease away, help you think clearly, steer off obesity, increase circulation, trigger that "feel good" hormone release, help lower blood pressure and cholesterol, improve self-confidence and flip on your optimism switch.

Physical exercise helps you to feel good about you and that's so critical when you are changing your health habits for the better. Less depression and anxiety are proven factors in people that exercise regularly. Add to that recovering faster from bodily injuries and life tragedy, which means exercise benefits you mind, body and soul.

So what is exercise?

It's the physical exertion of the body - forcing the body to perform physical activity which results in a healthy or healthier level of physical fitness both mentally and phys- ically.

Why Exercise?

* Build strong muscles
* Lose fat
* Increase metabolism
* Improve cardiovascular capacity
* Better sport performance
* Maintain bodyweight
* De-stress
* Improve social relations
* Improve cognitive ability
* Deter eating
* Better sex
* Helps elderly remain mobile and agile
* Increase energy
* Feel good

There are different levels of exercise and if you've just come off the couch you should always check with your doctor before boosting your heart rate and ALWAYS start slow, with light exercise until your systems get used to it.

Light Exercise - Is where you're still able to hold a con- versation with someone while exercising. Going for a brisk walk with a friend is a good example.

Moderate Exercise - This is where you are working your body a little harder, challenging it. You may get slightly out of breath with exercising at this level. Bringing your level up and down between light and moderate is incredibly effective, also referred to as interval training, where you're diversifying your heart rate and making your heart, lungs, mind and internal bodily systems keep guessing. Maximizing calories burned and removing boredom from the equation.

An example would be going for a bike ride at a good clip or maybe climbing up a hill. Leave the mountain for intense exercising.

Moderate exercising is where you should be at by at least the six week mark after beginning your exercise regimen.

Interesting Tidbit - Contrary to your belief, expert hunters and gatherers 25,000 years ago didn't exercise intensely every day, that's too hard on the body. They tried to minimize their physical exertion except for 2 days a week where they exercised intensely.

This gave the body time to physically recover, to stay strong and for energy reserves to be replenished when they really needed strong muscles and lungs to perform. Just think of how much mental and physical energy you'd need to hunt down an injured rhino or run from a hungry tiger that wants you for dinner!

Intense Exercise - Is where you are pushing your lungs and muscles close to their maximum capacity. We won't go further than that in this introductory book. Here you will have to concentrate on your breathing and will feel yourself tiring. Running, cycling hard, heavy weight training or intense book camp training sessions are good examples. This kind of exercise challenges your body and mind and ultimately should be incorporated into your routine about twice a week after you get rolling.

Both cardiovascular and muscle building are important in overall good health.

Cardiovascular exercise like cycling, running, swimming and tennis are aerobic activities that mean "with oxygen." This exercise is usually done at moderate levels for longer periods of time to burn energy. We used to be programmed that cardio was the best route to lose weight. Experts have changed their tune on this and now recommend muscle building combined with cardio exercise to maximize fat loss and keep it off.

Benefits of Cardio:

* Strengthens heart and lungs
* Lowers blood pressure and improves circulation
* Tones muscles and increases red blood cells, which carry more oxygen to muscles
* Improves sleep quality
* Reduces stress
* Betters mental health and self-confidence
* Triggers bone growth and strengthening
* Keeps muscles strong
* Improves endurance
* Improves life quality and quantity
* Triggers optimism

30-60 minutes aerobic activity 3-5 days a week minimum is recommended for good health.

In order to build fat burning lean muscle anaerobic exercise is required to build you bigger, leaner, stronger, and longer. Muscles are built and exercise hard for short times, a maximum of 2 minutes.

When exercising an aerobically, it's without oxygen to better muscle strength and quickness.

Anaerobic Exercise

* Sprinting
* Weight Lifting
* Interval Training
* Bursts of intense exercise like suicides or forced rep weight lifting

Anaerobic Benefits

* Strength gain
* Muscle building
* Increased bone strength
* Fast weight loss
* Helps keep weight off
* Strengthens joints and decreases injury

Disease

Obviously, disease is going to keep you from maintain an elite and optimally functioning mind and body. Years ago disease was thought of with more finality because they didn't have the modern medicines we do today to "cure" or at least minimize the symptoms of disease. In ancient times, many diseases meant the beginning of the end, often rapidly.

Times certainly have changed and with our technological advancements and more synthetic lifestyles we have created more disease or at least now how the tools to diagnose and recognize more of them. Disease will quickly steal from your quality of life, ranging in severity from mild with annoying symptoms like rashes and blisters, to severe where your respiratory system is challenged and even death may be the end result.

Prevention is the key in our world today and experts agree that it all starts with:

* Healthier eating
* Regular exercise
* More sleep
* Better lifestyles in general

In other words, disease prevention is multi-factorial and this means you are always going to have to juggle many balls if you want to maintain and strengthen your health and wellness.

Disease means an unhealthy disorder of the mind and body, often with pain and that interferes with the normal running of the bodily systems.

Degenerative muscle diseases like muscular dystrophies and lateral sclerosis, have distinct symptoms including:

* Walking Issues
* Decreased muscle strength
* Muscle fatigue
* Swallowing, chewing and speech problems
* Breathing issues

The bottom line is the majority of diseases we face today are linked with poor health choices that have manifested over time. Learning to make better food choices in the right amounts and right times, by exercising regularly and making better lifestyle choices, including improved sleep, you will help deter disease and improve your life quality.

Sleep

Don't you wish you could just sleep like a baby? Ever wonder why you can't?

As we grow interferences from all angles attack and infiltrate into our lives. We stop listening to our bodies and get up earlier and stay up later. We put harmful chemicals into our bodies that cause blockages in function.

Caffeine and alcohol are no-no's! We fill our systems full of nutrition-less processed and packaged high-fat, high-calories foods with emotional eating and very little or no exercise. This makes us fat and triggers disease like cardiovascular disease, diabetes, and obesity, which is linked to a huge array of serious diseases, inclusive of sleep apnea and snoring.

Sleep is also extremely important in good health. Your bodily systems need to shut down and recharge and sleep provide this opportunity. It's not just about getting 6-8 hours sleep each night because QUALITY of sleep is just as important. This means you aren't waking numerous times during the night because of controlled or uncontrolled circumstances. Many people have sleep issues that need professional attention. Problems like snoring, sleep apnea and night terrors are just a few problems that are directly connected to numerous other health problems.

Many people that snore and suffer from life-threatening sleep apnea are often obese. Having issues with hormone regulation because of excess fat is just the beginning. Often deciding to lose just a few pounds, can be the difference between sleeping and not getting the rest you need. I can't stress how important your health is when it comes to getting quality sleep. You can choose to ignore it and suffer or step up to the plate and deal with it head on.

That's not even getting into the psychology of it all, because obese people are more likely to be depressed and cause anxiety, emotional issues that just trigger more stress and overeating. The cycle is never ending and it all begins with poor eating and exercise habits.

Tips to Better Sleep

* Sleep Routine - By sticking to regular sleep/wake times you are teaching your body when it's time to shut down and wake up. We are creatures of habit and find comfort in routine. Having a schedule of sleep is going to give your body and mind the ability to have a quality sleep to recharge.

* Night time Ritual - Giving your body wind down time before bed is important. Maybe you want to turn the lights down and have a herbal cup of tea or read a book before bed. The idea is to signal to your internal systems you are getting ready to sleep.

* Limit Physical Activity - Near bedtime, you don' t want to rev your systems up. Getting your heart rate up by going to the gym or even dancing around the house means your endorphins are pumping and adrenaline, natural energy in your body is running full tilt. What this does, is signal to your body it's time to wake up and perform, not settle down for sleep. If you like to exercise later in the day make certain it's at least 2 hours prior to bedtime so you mental and physical have the chance to wind down.

Sleeping well is a part of this by establishing a healthy sleeping routine, one where you avoid stimulants like exercise and caffeine at night. Learn to relax and slow down each night. Lower the lights, turn the music down and do something relaxing like read a book or take a lukewarm bubble bath. Set your sleep and wake times and teach your body to get ready for sleep. In time with persistence, patience and continued smart health choices, you will move forward.

JUST DON'T QUIT!

Mental

So what is mental health?

It's essentially your overall attitude and approach to living your life. The physiological, genetic, environmental and psychological factors in life are all relevant in developing your mental.

Your mind is an EXTREMELY powerful thing. If you can "think" it you can do it.

Good mental health means you are free of depression and anxiety, over-stressing and worrying, addictions and various other psychological issues. Good mental health allows us to . . .

* Make better life choices
* Have healthy relationships at work and personally
* Improve overall physical health
* Deal better with life's curve balls
* Uncover your true potential
* View life optimistically rather than negatively and unproductively

Excess stress is a huge factor in mental health issues along with your nutritional and exercise habits. By losing weight and getting your body into shape physically, you will remove negative interference in your thinking. Being good to yourself and doing things that make you happy are a step in the right direction to great mental health.

Things like regular meditation, massage, saunas and other holistic treatments will help you naturally find your balance. This helps you to give you body a break, relax, unwind and rejuvenate. All of which are going to improve your mental life perspective and better your health as a whole.

Did you know . . . Happy people tend to have less body fat and are healthier in general than people with a negative life perspective? It does take more muscles to frown!

My Thoughts . . .

Each of these factors is going to determine your quality of life. It's a choice and by making the decision to better yourself in each of these areas. Get rid of the negative and make the positive habit, you're going to build your body lean and strong and send dangerous free-radicals packing sooner not later so disease doesn't manifest. Take this information, find what works for you and apply it.

Basic Causes of Interference in Good Health

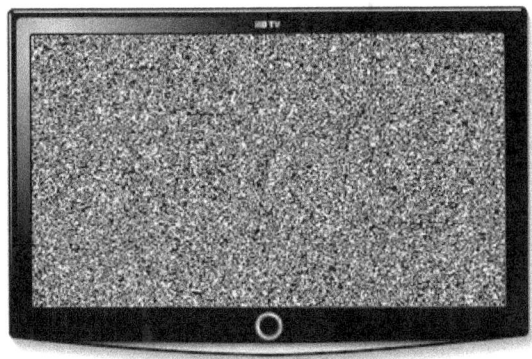

Every facet of life has a foundation for success and is-sues that keep that from happening. For instance, if you are trying to get an "A" on your test, you know you are going to have to study to get it. If you are feeling sick and aren't physically well enough to study, this will interfere with your results. If you overdose on caffeine, you might not be able to concentrate enough to get the desired re-sults. Maybe you pulled an all-nighter studying and can't stay awake to write the test.

The point is you can't succeed unless all the factors fall into place for you. The same applies with overall good health on a broader scale. There is no right or wrong here. It's just "better" for you, making better choices through trial and error you are going to figure out what works for you. Then you are going to fine-tune it some more and figure out a better choice.

Good health is something that is ALWAYS changing and ALWAYS will. It needs constant maintenance and monitoring and an open mind to make the changes that benefit YOU. The minute you understand and accept this you will be able to set yourself up for success always. It's a never-ending path to good health that isn't easy but is worth everything. YOU are worth it! Having your head on straight and taking care of your "mental" is a huge part of good health for the long run.

Interferences in Good Health

* Lack of Exercise

Solution - Turning back the clocks and getting back to the basics. Building your body leaner, bigger, stronger with regular challenging cardiovascular activity up to an hour 3-5 days a week, and muscle building/strength training 2-3 times a week for 15-20 minutes each session.

* Poor Eating Habits

Solution - Make the commitment to ditching the fast foods, highly processed and packaged treats and nutrition-less snacks and sugary sodas. Instead, fuel your body with lean meats, complex carbohydrates, plenty of fresh fruits and veggies, fatty fish and sparing amounts of healthy or unsaturated fats, giving your body the energy it needs to burn fat and the fuel required to function optimally.

* Lack of Sleep

Solution - Stop trying to convince yourself getting less sleep and more done is a good thing because it isn't. Instead commit to setting a bedtime and wakeup time and make it routine. Settle yourself down to sleep at night instead of getting stimulated and if you have sleep issues interfering get professional help. Often, losing weight by exercising and eating sensibly will do the trick. Make sure you get at least 7-8 hours quality sleep each night.

* Not Enough Sunlight

Solution - Make sure you get at least 15 minutes every day of unprotected sun exposure to get your dose of Vitamin D. If you can do this routinely in the morning first thing, you will set your internal biorhythm up for successful and productive function.

* Water Deprived

Solution - Your body and its systems can't function optimally without adequate water. If you find you are thirsty, you're already dehydrated. It's important you get at least 6-8 glasses of water a day and more if you are exercising. Carry a bottle of water around with you so you can think sharp, have ample energy stores and burn fat quickly.

* Stress/Mental
Solution - Taking the time to deal with stress instead of letting it bottle up inside is critical in good health. Exercise is an excellent form of de-stressing. It's something our ancestors did quite successfully. Actually, any sort of physical activity works, because what needs tending here is the natural intrinsic "fight or flight" response. Meditation and massage also works. Find ways that get rid of your stress and apply regularly. Positive thought and working towards this is also something is important in making sure you are mentally healthy.

* Good Hygiene

Solution - Many people don't realize that regular good hygiene practices are very important in maintaining good overall health, particularly in deterring disease. I don't think I need to go through these, but I will mention that regular hand washing is very important.

* Minimize Toxins

Solution - Eating organic, drinking clean water, staying away from environmental toxins, removing harmful chemicals from your household, are a few steps you can take to lowering your exposure to toxins and moving to cleaner, healthier living.

My Thoughts . . .

By recognizing and removing the negative life choices we make that interfere with poor health as a whole, we will help strengthen the mind and body, understanding that "healthy" is defined differently for each one of us. You may feel that eating right and exercising moderately 2-3 days a week with a fairly muscular body with a little extra fat is healthy for you. Another person may believe that taking the time to de-stress daily with meditation, eating vegetarian cuisine and training 5-6 days a week with high intensity is healthy.

THERE IS NO WRONG OR RIGHT HERE. What matters is that you figure out YOUR healthy and work towards it. In general, a bigger, leaner, stronger, longer body is the key.

Steps for Changes That Stick

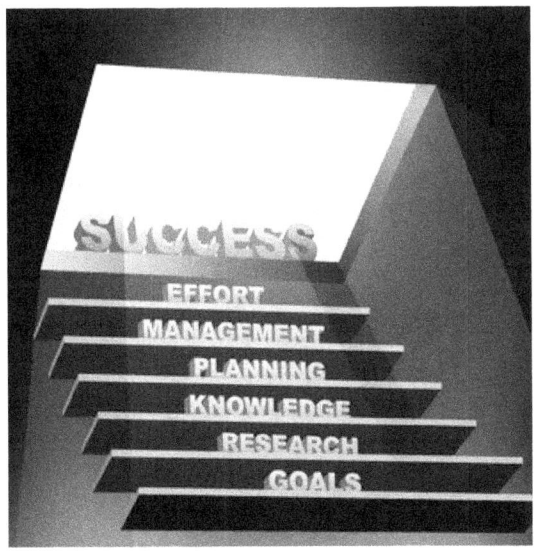

Before you make any plans for change, it's important we're clear on a few things. One is that if you are going to make changes in your life habits for the better it's important you set them up to stick for the long run.
Next, is that you understand if you want to make a change you are going to have to practice, practice, and practice a little more. Changes that stick are repeated and learned actions that eventually become habit. When they reach the "habit" mark, you have succeeded with the transformation.

So, if you want to switch your sugar loaded simple sugar white bread to nutrient dense, fiber rich and longer lasting whole grain bread, you are going to have to consciously make the switch and stick with it.

You might ease in, depending on your tolerances and preferences, with one slice unhealthy white bread and one slice healthy complex carbohydrate brown bread. In time, you'll switch this to two slices of the good stuff and keep repeating until you've made it a habit. It's something you prefer, enjoy, have developed a taste for and don't have to think about.

If you are truly looking to change your body, lifestyle or thinking for the better, for the purpose of improving your health, then try to understand the process is essentially the same.

Being Successful in Change Includes

ATTENTION FOCUSED - With change, you need to ac-tually think and perceive it to be possible and you'll look constantly for signs that are supporting our actions. The flip side is if you don't believe the change to be possible you will search and even create evidence to support this. YOUR FOCUS is your momentum. Believe you can do it, keep your focus and you will.

HABITS DAILY - If you are going to be successful in changing your comfortable behaviors you're going to have to change or alter your daily habits. This is a con-scious process that needs to be focused on and worked on until you add the new healthy habits you want and remove the ones you don't want. Let's say you are trying to build your lean muscle to help you burn more calories and zap fat always. This involves making smarter food choices and lifting weights regularly. Eating a slice of whole grain bread with peanut butter for breakfast in-stead of your usual packaged muffin is a great start.

Taking 15 minutes two days a week to focus on muscle building exercises is also a great new habit to help you reach your goal, instead of just sleeping in.

Your new daily habits are going to help propel you to your new healthy goals, but it's going to take persistence and effort. There is no other way, so either swallow that down or live under your true potential.

Relationships - These may also need to change depending on your goals. Perhaps you might have to stop hanging out with your overweight video "gamer" so much and create new relationships with people at the gym, that have the same life direction as you. When it comes to eating, you may be wise to stop partying with your friends every weekend and see if you can find a new healthier hobby where you connect with people that support a healthy lifestyle a little more. Maybe you'd like to try a rowing club or maybe a hiking group and find some relationships there.

Here are the basic steps for changes that stick.

Step One - Decide on Specifics

Here you need to decide specifically on what changes you're going to make. If you want to gain muscle and lose ten pounds of fat, that's what you need to write down. Maybe you want to add ten pounds of muscle or perhaps losing the nasty cigarette habit and cutting out processed foods are your goals.

The problem here is some people just really don't know what they want. They may want to get "healthy" and that's all great. If you don't know EXACTLY what results you want to see and how to get there it's really just a lot of stinky smoke blowing.

Step Two - Commit to Believing

Anyone can go through the motions or tell themselves something and just never follow through with it. Do yourself a favor and don't waste time. If you want to make a change you have to really WANT it and BELIEVE it. Dream about it, talk about it, and write about it. This will help you truly believe.

Step Three - Remind Yourself - Reinforce

Whether you have to write notes to yourself and stick them all over the house or have a friend ask you about it. You MUST reinforce what you are changing and why. Remind yourself of where you are and your final destination. This will help motivate, inspire and keep you focused on your goals.

Step Four - Reviewing Regularly

It's important to monitor your efforts towards your goals. Don't micro-manage yourself, but make sure you are consciously aware of your efforts. Maybe you will have a routine that you record in your journal each day. Go back through this daily to make sure you are doing what you intend.

Holding yourself accountable and teaching yourself to get used to these changes is only going to set you up for long-term success.

Step Five - Adjust

When you are making changes expect adjustments and adaptation to come with it. If you want to build a lean and sexy body and get up to hit the gym most mornings. Then you are going to have to adjust to the fact you are getting up earlier than you are conditioned for.

Expecting this and making the adjustment positively is going to help this transition of change smoother and less stressful, increasing your success conversion rate.

My Thoughts . . .

By taking the time to think through change before you begin, you're more likely to make effective changes that work for you and stick for the long run. Always keep the big picture in mind, be patient and make adjustments in your life you know make sense and will stick for the long run if you step them up for success.
Put your general knowledge of health and wellness, marry it with your personal preferences and tolerances, add a dash of logic, confidence, persistence and belief, this will make any change possible.

Strong Body Myths Gutted

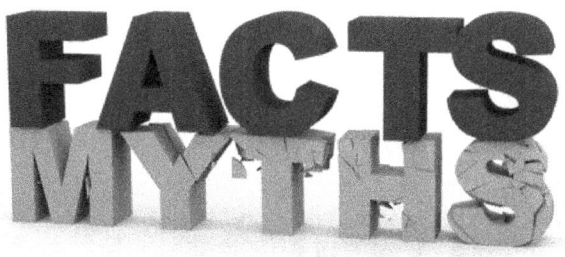

Fib 1 - Weight control and good health depends only on counting calories

Truth: Calories going into your body does not equal calories going out. Of course eating less calories, while still giving your body what it requires, can help you lose weight, not every food is processed the same. Just think about eating a bag of potato chips and a sweet potato equal in calories. Sure you are taking in the same amount of calories with each, but your physical and emotional responses will be very different. The simple processed sugars and unhealthy saturated fats from the chips will shoot your blood sugars through the roof quickly, leaving you with a depressing crash shortly after and no nutritional gain.

The sweet potato is a complex carbohydrate loaded with long-term energy, fiber, lots of nutrients and stays level with your blood sugars. It's the same calories, but two very different foods and outcomes.

Fib 2 - You'll ruin your eyes reading with very little light

Truth: This one is an old wives tale. Specialists agree that reading in dim light isn't going to negatively affect your eyes physically, although it may cause strain and squinting. Wonder if it's true that squinting causes wrinkles?

Fib 3 - Poor you - slow metabolism causes obesity

Truth: Nice excuse, but it just doesn't cut it. Excess weight is caused by lack of physical exertion and not because of slower metabolisms. Experts believe that unwanted weight gain comes from poor eating choices, lack of exercise and numerous other mental and emotional issues that often are associated with being overweight and unhealthy.

Fib 4 - If you don't wear a hat you're going to lose more heat through your head

Truth: This is another old wives tale. Scientists have found that you aren't going to lose heat faster through your head than any other part of your body. If you aren't wearing gloves on a cold day just as much heat can escape through your hands.

Fib 5 - Training with weights will make fat into lean muscle

Truth: This one is physiologically impossible because they are two completely different substances. It's like comparing apples to oranges. Now weights or strength training will help to build muscle and this triggers a metabolic speed up and fat burning is a part of this, although this isn't an absolute relationship. If you want to build lean muscle weight training is very important along with making better food choices and cardio exercise. Think of it as a multi-factorial issue.

My Thoughts . . .
Getting to the truth of the myth is important when you are looking to take action and transform your body bigger, leaner, stronger, and longer. If something every sounds too good to be true it probably is. Get to the bottom of your skepticism and make sure you've the whole fact before you take the first step. Information is knowledge and knowledge is power but it needs to be factual to matter.

How to Get the Body You Want

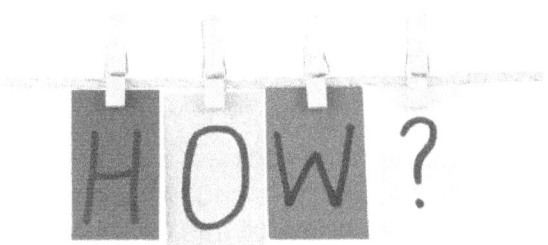

The first thing you have to do is decide what kind of body you want. Just look back a few chapters if you need help setting up and figuring out your goal changes.

Do you want to build lots of beautiful lean muscle, zap fat and lose weight?

Do you want to gain weight and strength by building muscle?

Do you want to get lean and strong and maximize your calorie burn?

WHAT DO YOU WANT?

For the sake of numbers and popularity let's just say you want to build lean muscle, firm and tone your body and lose fat for the long run.

Here's how you can do just that.

* Eat less calories than your body is expending. The best way to do this is a combination of eating less and exercising more. Eating less might now even be a matter of eating less but eating smarter. By choosing to eat a balanced diet of organic lean protein, complex carbs, plenty of fruits and veggies and lots of water, you can eliminate oodles of unnecessary bad fats and calories from your diet if you are accustomed to eating processed, packed and "fast" foods.

Simply making better food choices, will often lower your overall calorie intake and help you lose weight.
By adding regular exercising to this, is also going to help boost your metabolism or the rate you burn calories and zap fat faster. When your heart, lungs and internal systems are working harder, your body is expending more energy as a whole.

* Exercise smart. By incorporating regular intense exercise into your day you're going to help your body metabolize fat and build lean muscle. Remembering the more lean muscle you build the more calories you are going to burn even when snoozing. Fat burns less calories than muscle.

Most experts recommend a combination of cardiovascular exercise and weight training or strength training. At least 45 minutes cardiovascular exercise 3-5 days a week and weight training 2-3 times a week for 15 minutes is a great start. This will help your body to build lean muscle, burn fat and get strong.

NOTE - You have to eat if you want to burn fat and build lean muscle. If you aren't giving your body enough calories and protein to build muscle you are just going to burn it. When exercising regularly you need at least 2-3 servings of lean protein, along with well balanced eating, to give your body the tools to build lean muscle for you. The more you are weight training and building muscle the more healthy food choices you're going to have to eat. Making sure before and after your training you enjoy a snack of healthy carbs and lean protein to replenish and help your body recover. Working with a fitness trainer to learn the ropes is an excellent idea, particularly when starting.

* Remove negative lifestyle habits. If you are looking to get your body into wonderful shape you're going to need energy to do this. If you smoke, drink and do drugs you are steeling not only your precious brain cells, but also the energy you need to train. Poisoning your body knowingly just doesn't make sense. If you really want to quit you can. Believe it and get to the process of making it happen. This is only going to help you reach your personal health and wellness goals faster.

* Sleep is critical in all good health. If you are working hard to build your body strong you are especially going to need quality sleep. If you want to maximize your muscle gain and weight loss your body has to rest, repair and restore. There are no exceptions to the rules here. If you aren't sleeping, your body is not gaining strength as it should and you aren't maximizing your efforts. 6-8 hours sleep each night is a must, more if you are training hard.

* Your mental is a huge factor in your success. The mind is a powerful thing and if you want to reach your goals of muscle building, disease prevention and weight loss you are going to have to be on board with your brain. Make sure you take time to treat your mental. Perhaps taking a few minutes each day to meditate and calm yourself will help you get healthier faster. Some find that just taking a walk by the lake or having a massage regularly is enough

to get their head in a happy place and better able to han-
dle life stresses. Make sure you do this because your
head is critical is success.

* Eating organic will help make certain you are minimiz-
ing harmful toxins from pesticides, hormones and the
environment from entering your system and interfering
with healthy function.

Next I'm going to give you a sample of an exercise and
eating regimen for an average woman, just so you can
have an idea of what a healthy eating and exercise plan
might look like with the goals of losing fat and building
lean and sexy muscle.

Sample Meal Day

Breakfast
2 poached eggs
1 piece whole grain toast
1/2 cup low-fat yogurt
1 cup fresh berries
Water
Calories . . .450

Lunch
1 cup couscous
1 cup fresh vegetables
2 cups spinach, 1/2 cups carrots, 1/2 cup cucumbers, 1/2
cup tomatoes, 1/2 cup peppers, 1/4 slivered almonds,
drizzle salad dressing
1 piece fresh fruit
Green Tea
Water
Calories . . . 450

Dinner

Grilled chicken breast
Sweet potato - baked
1 cup grilled asparagus
1 cup streamed broccoli
Water
Calories . . . 500

Snacks
5-6 whole grain crackers with 1 tbsp peanut butter
Orange
1 cup pudding

Overview
This is a start and what you need to do is personalize it.
2-3 servings of protein
4-6 breads and cereals
5-7 servings of fruits and vegetables
2-3 servings of good fat

Sample Exercise Day

Cardio

Approximately 45 minutes biking, hiking, running, fast
walking, aerobic exercise, cross training, tennis, etc.
What's important is that you work at your own pace and
make certain you challenge yourself. If you are at least
breaking a light sweat then you are working your body
hard.

Weight/Strength Training

Weight machines in the gym are a great way to build your
strength. With the machines you're less likely to injure
yourself versus using free weights. Always work with an
expert trainer until you learn the ropes or you can seri-
ously hurt yourself.

With strength training you can do a combination of sit-ups, lunges, squats, pushups and "burpees" to start. Of course stretching is important BEFORE and AFTER any exercising.

Note - Interval training is the best exercise option for getting results fast. An example might be to bike at a moderate pace for 10 minutes, push yourself for 2 minutes and then settle back down to a moderate pace. By changing your intensity level regularly you are going to challenge your body to burn more calories and you aren't going to get bored. Boot camp training sessions are excellent for building lean muscle and zapping fat fast, alternating periods of high intensity cardio with low intensity cardio and various degrees of weight training and strength training in between.

My Thoughts . . .

You can get the body you want just as long as you first figure out what you want. Then gather the information you need to make it happen. Finally applying this knowledge, stick to it, adjust as needed and DO NOT QUIT. You are important and so is your health.

Final Words

You're Only Human - Right?

Don't get discouraged when you trip and fall or slip off track occasionally. This doesn't mean you've failed it just means you are human. Maybe you want to get your body muscular, lean and strong for swimsuit season a few months away. It's tough not to get discouraged when you go away on vacation and don't exercise and eat like it was your last supper for the whole week, only to come back to reality and realize you've gained ten pounds and it's not muscle!

SO WHAT???
You are human and you can't change the past. The right thing to do is let it go and pick up where you left off. Is it going to be tough initially? Yes! Are you going to feel like just throwing in the towel? It wouldn't be normal not to. The choice is yours. You can persevere and commit to good health choices for the long run, through thick and thin, or you can just exist always knowing there is a whole lot more happiness in you that you just don't feel you are deserved of.

Applying the 4 Hour Body Plus concept is going to give you the "know-how" to get your health right where you want it.

Change is tough.
Losing weight is tough.
Muscle building is tough.
Making your new lifestyle habits stick for life is very tough.

FACT

You control you. If you want to change your body, mind and overall quality and longevity of life for the better, then you need to make the decision and commitment to make it happen.

There is no perfect diet, eating strategy or weight loss program out there for everyone. What you need to do is take from your knowledge and life experiences what works for you, then apply and adjust as you learn new information and make better life choices to help you reach your personal goals.

Your health is the most important asset you have. If you care about you it's a no-brainer you are always going to strive to build your body and mind stronger to serve you better for the long run.

Experts agree the way people used to live thousands of years ago makes sense. Of course, it's not practical to-day, but we can take from this what we know and apply. Eating natural foods is going to fuel your body right, lean proteins to burn fat and provide energy, goods carbs that will give your body the fiber and nutrients it needs to naturally purge toxins and run smoothly. Vitamins and minerals from healthy fruits and veggies and nuts is going to satisfy all your other nutritional requirements, helping your internal systems give you the energy and mental ability to function optimally.

Time for you to put on your positive cap, open your mind and get started. Just put one foot in front of the other all eyes forward. You WILL get there. The first step is actually BELIEVING!

We have the choice to look for the positive or the negative in life. You can choose to lift someone up or to stomp on them. Writing is my passion and I work hard at it, with the goal of helping make people better. If you gain a new piece of knowledge, read something that makes you think, or perhaps even smile a few times, then I am happy and content!

Life's just too short not to tune into optimism. If your glass is half full, then I invite you to read my writing, and if you have a minute to spare when you're through, **I would appreciate your review.** This will help me better myself and my writing. I thank you in advance and appreciate you.